# Simple Things Matter

## Your Personal Guide to Wellness

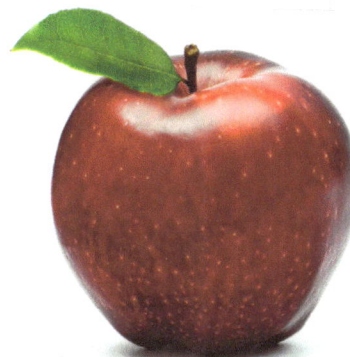

"Wellness" is a simple but powerful way of being. Being "well" means many things to many individuals, but ultimately wellness is the maintenance of good health and the adoption of healthy behaviors to get and stay healthy.

Genetic predisposition to certain illness accounts for less than 5% of chronic disease. Seventy-five percent of chronic illnesses such as Diabetes, Heart Disease and some forms of cancer are totally preventable with simple lifestyle and behavior change.[1] That's right, preventable. The things that you do (lifestyle) and the way in which you engage in your lifestyle (behaviors) are the keys to preventing or delaying the onset of illness or disease. This means that YOU are in complete control of your health.

Wellness is about choosing lifestyles and behaviors that promote optimal health—physically, mentally, socially and even spiritually. In order to be well, you must actively ENGAGE in activities that will support your health and ensure that you achieve the highest quality of life. Choosing lifestyles and behaviors that are focused on your well being will help you enjoy life to the fullest.

Individuals who make unhealthy lifestyle choices may end up with chronic, debilitating disease and illness that can cost you and others considerable healthcare dollars. Americans spend more than $240 billion each year to treat chronic disease and illness, such as diabetes, obesity, and tobacco related disease; all of these conditions can be effectively managed, reduced or even prevented with simple lifestyle and behavior choices that promote well-being.[2]

The most important motivator for choosing a healthy lifestyle should be the fact that you are improving the length and quality of your life. You owe it to yourself and to your family to change behavior.

The next sections will provide you with simple solutions that promote wellness and overall good health. This booklet is meant to be a guide to support your personal journey and just touches on some of the primary prevention aspects of good health and well-being.

For further information about the StayFit™ Plan program, log on to Simplicity Health Plan's website at www.simplicityhealthplans.com and enjoy all of the free programs, resources and tools designed to help you stay healthy and well. (You must be a StayFit™ Plan member to access the StayFit™ Plan resources).

# Simple Solutions
## To Staying Healthy

Research has shown that even the most modest changes in your nutritional habits and physical activity can have a profound impact on your overall well-being.

Good health is not a guarantee, but YOU can make better lifestyle and behavior choices that will improve your chances of staying healthy.

There are several immediate steps that you can take to begin your personal path to wellness.

1. Be sure to receive your annual preventive exams. Preventive exams include important screenings depending on your age and gender.[3] Individual factors will also determine what types of screenings are ordered by your personal physician. Preventive exams are important because they can detect early signs and/or symptoms of chronic disease that may be delayed or prevented through early treatment and interventions.

2. "You are what you eat." The rate of obesity in America is out of control. The most recent report shows that roughly 63% of the adult population in the United States is either overweight or obese and this number continues to rise.[4] Proper nutrition and portion control are foundational principals for maintaining proper weight and good health. Understanding which foods to eat and in what quantity is important to preventing many chronic diseases caused by being overweight.

3. Maintaining a healthy weight is vital to well-being. Obesity is linked to Type II Diabetes, Heart Disease, High Blood Pressure, Osteoarthritis and many other ailments[5]; and generally, controlling appetite and selecting a healthful diet that includes the appropriate amount of fats, carbohydrates (sugars), fiber and minerals to support the maintenance of individual weight.

4. Be active. Your body craves exercise and movement. Physical activity promotes brain health and helps to improve your mood as well as helps maintain strong bones.[6] A balance of activities such as walking, swimming, bicycling or jogging at least 30 minutes a day every day of the week is a great exercise regiment. Simple tasks such as housecleaning and mowing the lawn (not a riding mower) are also great ways to include physical activity into your daily routine.

5. Don't Smoke! Smoking poses serious health risks and has been directly correlated with cancer. Nicotine is a very addicting drug and makes it very difficult to quit smoking. The bottom line is that you are exposing yourself and others (secondhand smoke) to deadly toxins that will ultimately result in a costly chronic disease or death.[7] Resolve to quit today!

6. Personal safety is often overlooked as a way to maintain health and well-being. There are very simple and easy things you can do to ensure you do as much as you can to reduce your risk of avoidable accidents.

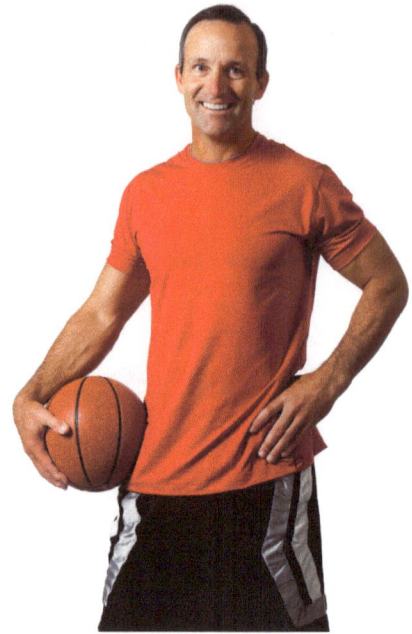

# Adult Preventive Guidelines

The grid below outlines the United States Preventive Service Task Force (USPSTF)[8] recommendations for Adult Preventive Screenings. The screenings are based on gender and age and are meant as a guide only. Be sure to see your personal care physician and/or healthcare provider regularly who will determine, along with you, the need for any additional exams and screenings based on your physical examination and family history.

| Adult Preventative Screening Guidelines | | | | | |
|---|---|---|---|---|---|
| Screening | Gender | Age 18-35 | Age 40-49 | Age 50-64 | Age 65+ |
| Blood Pressure | Male/Female | Annually<br>Normal <120/80<br>Pre-hypertension 120-139/80-89<br>Hypertension > 140/190 | | | |
| Lipids | Male/Female | Non-fasting total cholesterol and HDL-cholesterol beginning at age 35 for men and age 45 for women, repeat every 5 years.<br>(A fasting lipid profile should be done if total cholesterol > 200 (elevated cholesterol may not be a risk factor for heart disease) | | | |
| Colonoscopy | Male/Female | | | Fecal occult blood annually for age > 50.<br>Sigmoidoscopy or colonoscopy screening at age 50. | |
| Immunizations | Male/Female | Td or Tdap every 10 years<br><br>Varicella<br><br>Gardasil (HPV) Females 9 - 26 | Td or Tdap every 10 years | Influenza yearly**<br><br>Zostavak (shingles) after turning age 60<br><br>Td or Tdap every 10 years | Pneumococcal<br><br>Td or Tdap every 10 years |
| Pelvic & Pap | Female | Begin within 3 years of onset of sexual activity/no later than age 21.<br>Pap test yearly (or every 3 years after having three yearly normal Pap tests). Stops at age 65 unless high risk (previous positive Pap tests or previous Cervical Cancer). | | | |
| Mammogram | Female | | Every 1-2 years | Every 1-2 years | Every 1-2 years |
| Chlamydia | Female | All sexually active females younger than 25 years of age and all pregnant females at increased risk. | | | |
| Hepatitis B | Female | All pregnant females at first prenatal visit. | | | |
| Osteoporosis | Female | | | | Screen all women > 65 years of age, at-risk women > 60 years |

Source: http://www.uspreventiveservicestaskforce.org/adjultrec.htm

*\*\* The Flu Vaccine may not be necessary although it is recommended by the CDC. If you take the Flu Vaccine we recommend that you take it from a single dose vial. The single-dose units are made without thimerosal (thimerosal contains Mercury in very small amounts) as a preservative because they are intended to be opened and used only once. Additionally, the live-attenuated version of the vaccine (the nasal spray vaccine), is produced in single-dose units and does not contain thimerosal.*

# Eating Wisely

## Choosing a Healthy Diet

Your body depends on the foods you consume for energy, strength and physical fitness. Eating a variety of healthful natural foods ensures that you receive the best possible nutrition, including essential vitamins, minerals and fiber.[9] Processed foods are not natural foods and contain large amounts of omega-6 oils (vegetable, soybean, corn and sunflower oil), which in large quantities are not good for your health. Use virgin olive oil instead. Unfortunately Americans have been lead astray by the faulty thinking that you should have a diet low in fat and high in polyunsaturated fats and carbohydrates. The contrary is true. Diets containing normal amounts of saturated fats that are low in carbohydrates are actually better for you. *(see The Myth of Cholesterol)*

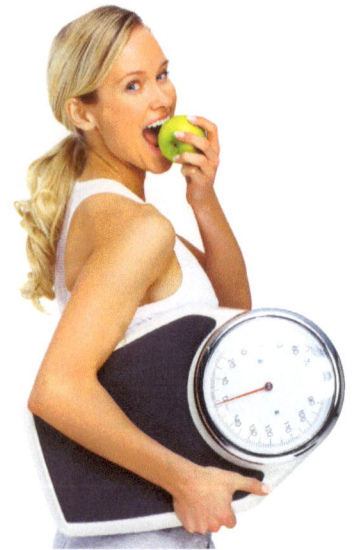

The American Diabetic Association (ADA) describes eating a variety of complex carbohydrates and a moderate amount of protein and fat as the key to healthy eating and weight control.[10] A balanced diet does not have to take a lot of effort. In fact, eating healthy is fairly simple if you incorporate these five simple eating principles:

1.  Portion size matters!  Today's portion sizes have grown up to 2-3 times the amount of food needed and/or required to make up a single portion size.[11] To guide your portion control, here are a few tips to adjust your nutritional intake to a correct portion size:
    a.  3 oz. of lean meat is equivalent to a deck of playing cards.
    b.  1 cup serving is about the size of a tennis ball.
    c.  1 oz. of a serving is equivalent to four dice.
    d.  1 tsp of a serving is equivalent to one die.
    e.  1 piece of fruit should fit in the palm of your hand.

2.  Use virgin olive oil and select dairy products, which will provide you with calcium and vitamins that your body needs. Butter is ok in moderate amounts. The ratio of omega-6 to omega-3 oils should be no more than 3:1 Eating processed foods may spike this ratio to 30:1 (not good).

3.  Reduce your intake of salts and sugars. Increased sodium (salt) increases your risk for developing high blood pressure.[12] Foods high in sugar are generally high in calories. High sugar diets are full of immediately available calories and if not used by your body within 2 hours are usually stored as fat and contribute to weight gain and associated disease. In addition, a diet high in sugar promotes tooth decay. Eating lots of carbohydrates without exercise will make you fat. Too many carbohydrates are the main cause of our increasingly overweight and obese population. Use salt with iodine, eat fish or take a vitamin with iodine to prevent thyroid problems.

4.  Include a variety of complex carbohydrates in your diet in moderation. These are found in whole grain breads, brown rice, beans and vegetables, which provide the fiber and nutrients that are required to maintain a healthy and well balanced diet. These select foods outweigh the limited nutritional benefits from simple carbohydrates such as white bread, processed foods, salty foods and sweet snacks.

5.  Count your calories. Counting your calories is just as important as ensuring the right portion control. Even some of the healthiest foods can be high in calories. To determine your caloric intake, use the health and wellness calculators in the StayFit™ Plan wellness resources located on the Simplicity Health Plans website at www.simplicityhealthplans.com. (You must be a StayFit™ Plan member to access the StayFit™ Plan resources)

# Eating Wisely

## Choosing a Healthy Diet

One of the biggest myths in America today is that you get fat from eating fat. Well, this is not entirely true. You get fat from eating too many carbohydrates (sugar) and not using the sugar within several hours after consumption. Most fat is not absorbed by your body.

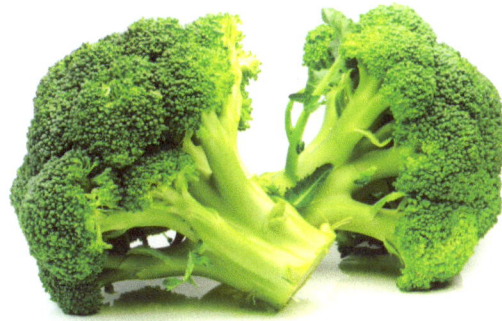

Carbohydrates are another fancy name for sugar. Most of the carbohydrates in your diet come from plant foods, such as grains, fruits, vegetables, legumes and nuts. The main role of carbohydrates is to provide your body with energy, which is primarily in the form of a sugar called glucose. Different types of carbohydrates are categorized based on the amount of sugar molecules that they contain. Simple carbohydrates are those that contain only one or two sugar molecules. Complex carbohydrates are those that contain more than two sugar molecules linked together. Carbohydrates are sugars like sucrose (plain table sugar) and fructose and glucose (sugars found in fruits and plants) all are used by your body to produce readily available energy. An orange has as much sugar as a can of cola. Fruit is loaded with sugar, so don't eat too much fruit. High fructose corn syrup is sugar just like any other sugar. It's only bad for you if you eat too much of it and don't use the energy it supplies.

Essentially you consume carbohydrates for energy. If the energy goes unused, the ingested sugar (carbohydrate) is converted and stored as fat. Americans eat and drink way too much sugar and exercise way too little. The plain and simple fact is that Americans are becoming overweight and obese from consuming too many carbohydrates (sugar) and not exercising. The result; stored excess fat that contributes to a growing waistline and creating a further barrier to exercise. All of this places individuals at risk for very serious chronic medical conditions like diabetes, heart disease, hypertension and some cancers. Fortunately, you CAN prevent these conditions by reducing the amounts of carbohydrates in your diet and getting enough exercise.

Sensible carbohydrate (sugar) intake is essential to overall good health, well-being and a slim waistline. The allowable daily amount of sugar is 7 teaspoons for women and 9 teaspoons for men.[13] However, today most Americans are consuming 10-20 times the allowable daily amount. In fact, if you drink one soda a day or eat one orange you are consuming about 16 teaspoons of sugar.

It is extremely important to eat a balanced diet that includes fats and carbohydrates in moderation. Be sure to incorporate exercise into your daily life. Try to "do" something immediately after you eat so that your body uses the energy that you just put into it such as go for a walk. This simple action could have a major impact on your body's ability to burn the carbohydrates you just consumed.

For sensible eating tips as well as diet tools, resources and recipes to help you maintain or improve your diet, log on to the StayFit™ Plan program at www.simplicityhealthplans.com (You must be a StayFit™ Plan member to access the StayFit™ Plan resources).

# Managing Your Weight

## Diet and Exercise

The Center for Disease Control and Prevention estimates that over 60% of the adult population and 31% of children are overweight or obese.[14] Recent data obtained by MRI in 2012, suggests that 63% of the US population is obese.

Being overweight contributes to many types of costly chronic disease. Overweight is defined as a body mass index (BMI) of 25-30 and obese is defined as a body mass index of greater than 30.[15] However, recent data suggests that a BMI of 28 or greater defines obesity.

While there are countless books, programs and medications available to help individual's lose weight the only true solution is burning more calories than you consume—diet and exercise.

Use the tips for eating wisely and facts about carbohydrates to help you understand about the things you can do to maintain or improve your diet, then engage in the weight management and diet tools, resources and programs on the StayFit™ Plan website to begin your journey to a healthy waistline.

Remember; be sure to pay particular attention to portion control and calorie counts. Incorporate physical activity into your daily routine. If you are just starting out, be sure to add activities slowly and incrementally allowing your body to adjust to your new routine. Most experts recommend that adults achieve at least 30 minutes of physical activity per day. Always check with your healthcare provider or personal physician before beginning a physical activity program.

### Setting a Goal

The most successful way to sustained weight loss is through slow and gradual weight loss that equates to one half pound to two pounds per week.[16] Rapid weight loss can actually be dangerous to your health and also has been shown to cause the "yo-yo" weight loss effect.[17] Research has shown that losing as little as 5-10% of your weight can reduce your risk of developing high blood pressure, high cholesterol and diabetes.

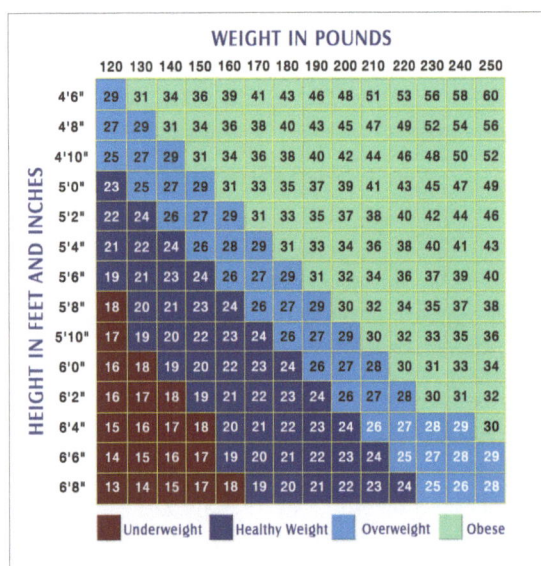

**WEIGHT IN POUNDS**

| HEIGHT IN FEET AND INCHES | 120 | 130 | 140 | 150 | 160 | 170 | 180 | 190 | 200 | 210 | 220 | 230 | 240 | 250 |
|---|---|---|---|---|---|---|---|---|---|---|---|---|---|---|
| 4'6" | 29 | 31 | 34 | 36 | 39 | 41 | 43 | 46 | 48 | 51 | 53 | 56 | 58 | 60 |
| 4'8" | 27 | 29 | 31 | 34 | 36 | 38 | 40 | 43 | 45 | 47 | 49 | 52 | 54 | 56 |
| 4'10" | 25 | 27 | 29 | 31 | 34 | 36 | 38 | 40 | 42 | 44 | 46 | 48 | 50 | 52 |
| 5'0" | 23 | 25 | 27 | 29 | 31 | 33 | 35 | 37 | 39 | 41 | 43 | 45 | 47 | 49 |
| 5'2" | 22 | 24 | 26 | 27 | 29 | 31 | 33 | 35 | 37 | 38 | 40 | 42 | 44 | 46 |
| 5'4" | 21 | 22 | 24 | 26 | 28 | 29 | 31 | 33 | 34 | 36 | 38 | 40 | 41 | 43 |
| 5'6" | 19 | 21 | 23 | 24 | 26 | 27 | 29 | 31 | 32 | 34 | 36 | 37 | 39 | 40 |
| 5'8" | 18 | 20 | 21 | 23 | 24 | 26 | 27 | 29 | 30 | 32 | 34 | 35 | 37 | 38 |
| 5'10" | 17 | 19 | 20 | 22 | 23 | 24 | 26 | 27 | 29 | 30 | 32 | 33 | 35 | 36 |
| 6'0" | 16 | 18 | 19 | 20 | 22 | 23 | 24 | 26 | 27 | 28 | 30 | 31 | 33 | 34 |
| 6'2" | 16 | 17 | 18 | 19 | 21 | 22 | 23 | 24 | 26 | 27 | 28 | 30 | 31 | 32 |
| 6'4" | 15 | 16 | 17 | 18 | 20 | 21 | 22 | 23 | 24 | 26 | 27 | 28 | 29 | 30 |
| 6'6" | 14 | 15 | 16 | 17 | 19 | 20 | 21 | 22 | 23 | 24 | 25 | 27 | 28 | 29 |
| 6'8" | 13 | 14 | 15 | 17 | 18 | 19 | 20 | 21 | 22 | 23 | 24 | 25 | 26 | 28 |

Underweight  Healthy Weight  Overweight  Obese

Generally, a diet high in vegetables and lean meat like chicken, turkey and fish is very good for controlling and maintaining your weight. Don't forget to take a good multivitamin every so often; once a day may not be required.

Body Mass Index (BMI) is a relative measure of weight management and can be a helpful tool for individuals who are trying to maintain or lose weight. A healthy BMI is 18.5 to 25. Use the chart to find your BMI.

# Get Active

## Incorporating Physical Activity

The importance of physical activity is paramount to achieving physical and emotional well-being which ultimately contributes to overall good health. Regular physical activity can help reduce or eliminate the unnecessary health risks associated with physical inactivity. The latest information shows that inactivity among Americans remains relatively high, and therefore predisposes individuals to a host of chronic illness. [18]

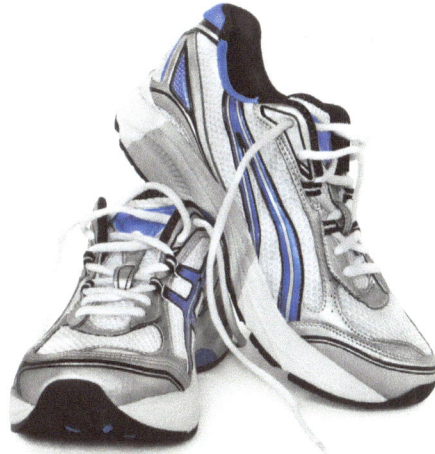

For all individuals, some activity is better than none. Physical activity is safe for almost everyone, and the health benefits of physical activity far outweigh the risks.

Adults ages 18-64 should do at least 3 hours a week of moderate-intensity activities or at least 1 hour a week of vigorous-intensity aerobic physical activity. Moderate-intensity physical activity includes activities that incorporate at least 30 minutes of cardiovascular activity 3 times per week and vigorous-intensity includes activities that incorporate at least 45-60 minute of cardiovascular activity 5-6 times per week.[19] A combination of moderate- and vigorous-intensity activity is optimal to maintaining overall physical health. Additional health benefits may be achieved by increasing physical activity to 5 hours a week of moderate-intensity aerobic physical activity, or 2 hours a week of vigorous-intensity physical activity, or an equivalent combination of both. The best way to sustain a physical activity in your life is to incorporate activities that you enjoy so that you will continue to engage in them and not get bored.

Building strong bones is important too. Adults should incorporate muscle-strengthening activities that involve all major muscle groups at least 2 days per week or more. In addition, individuals who engage in regular physical activity sleep better and have improved emotional well-being.

The health benefits of physical activity include a lower risk of early death, heart disease, stroke, Type 2 diabetes, high blood pressure, decrease cholesterol levels, metabolic syndrome, colon and breast cancers, prevention of weight gain, weight loss when combined with diet, improved cardio- respiratory and muscular fitness. [20]

StayFit™ Plan offers you a variety of online resources, programs and tools to help get you started on a physical activity program that's right for you. You even have access to a personal health coach, blogs, social networks and other resources that provide you suggestions, support and motivation on your path to physical fitness. Don't wait another day, log on to the StayFit™ Plan website at www.simplicityhealthplans.com to get started today!

# Quit Smoking

## Kick Your Tobacco Habit

One hundred thirty five million adults ages 20-64 are currently employed in the United States and of those adults, 23% are current smokers. [21]

Smoking causes a variety of diseases and cancers and is basically a slow way to die. One in two lifetime smokers will die from their habit.[22]

Half of these deaths will occur in middle age. The mixture of nicotine and carbon monoxide in each cigarette you smoke temporarily increases your heart rate and blood pressure, consequently straining your heart and blood vessels.

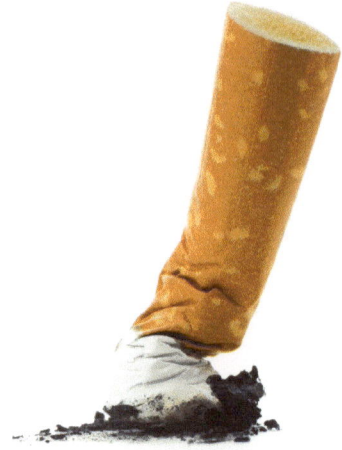

Clearly the ill effects of tobacco use are alarming, yet interestingly enough, most of these conditions can be reversed or delay the onset of disease by "kicking the habit".

Thankfully, when you stop smoking, the body experiences positive side effects and begins to repair itself rather quickly; the healing process begins within just 20 minutes of quitting. Refer to the smoking cessation time line table on the next page to see how quickly your body begins to repair itself.

### Quick Tips to Smoking Cessation

There is no single solution to help an individual quit smoking. The universal truth is that YOU must want to quit. Quitting smoking is one of the best lifestyle choices you can make to promote your personal well being. Below are a few helpful tips that can place you on a path to a tobacco free life.

- Set a quit date. Try and choose a date that will be stress free and one where you will most likely succeed.
- Be sure and speak with your physician, especially if you have health problems and are concerned about issues such as weight gain.
- Find a partner or a champion. Someone who can go on the quit journey with you and is willing to be your personal quit coach. Tell your family and friends about your intentions and ask them for their support throughout your process.
- Know your triggers! Pinpoint when you desire your cigarette most and do your best to avoid or eliminate these triggers. Think about alternative activities you can engage in that will take your mind off of smoking when you feel the "urge". Remember, in most cases, your craving will only last for 3-5 minutes at a time.
- Be positive and confident you can quit. Believe in yourself and you will be able to accomplish your goal.

# Smoking Cessation Timeline

The best time to quit smoking is right now. Yes, quitting can be difficult, but the benefits to your health can begin in as little as 20 minutes.

The timeline below shows you what happens to your body when you quit smoking.

| Timeline | What Happens to Your Body When You Quit Smoking |
| --- | --- |
| 20 minutes | Blood pressure and pulse return to normal. |
| 8 hours | Oxygen levels return to normal. Nicotine and carbon monoxide levels in blood reduced by half. |
| 12 hours | Carbon monoxide levels in blood drop to normal. |
| 24 hours | Carbon monoxide will be eliminated from the body. Lungs start to clear out mucous and other tobacco debris. |
| 48 hours | There is no nicotine left in the body. Ability to taste and smell begins to improve greatly. |
| 72 hours | Breathing becomes easier. Bronchial tubes begin to relax and energy levels increase. |
| 2-12 weeks | Circulation improves. Lung function increases. |
| 3-9 months | Coughing, wheezing and breathing problems improve as lung functions are increased by up to 10%. |
| 12 months | Excess risk of coronary heart is reduced by about half and declines gradually hereafter. |
| 5 years | Risk of heart attack falls to about half that of a smoker, Risk of stroke returns to the level who have never smoked (5 - 15 years). |
| 10 - 15 years | Risk of lung cancer is reduced to close to that observed in nonsmokers. Risk of coronary heart disease falls to the same as someone who has never smoked. If you have quit smoking before age 50, you have halved the risk of dying in the next 15 years compared with continuing smokers. |

# Personal Safety

## Simple Things to Prevent Injury

Often we go through our days engaged in everyday tasks, such as driving, housework, spending time with friends and family, taking personal safety and well being for granted.

There are a lot of simple things that you can do to prevent illness, injury and accidents from occurring throughout your lifetime.

Some of this information may be familiar to you and some of it may be enlightening. Either way, it is always important to adopt and engage in behaviors and lifestyles that will promote the highest level of personal safety and wellness.

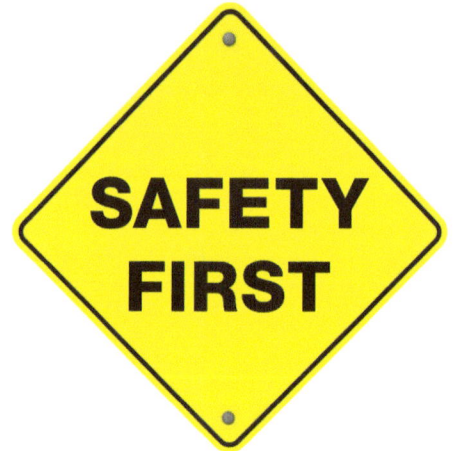

1. Drink plenty of clean water. (See water consumption)
2. Eat healthy non-processed foods. (Do not overeat)
3. Do not smoke.
4. Wear a seat belt when driving in a car.
5. Drive a car with air bags.
6. Stay as active as possible.
7. Get your preventive care and screenings on time.
8. Take a multivitamin occasionally. Everyday is not necessary. Think about incorporating supplement tablets such as B12 if you do not eat a lot of meat. Do not take mega doses of vitamins as they can harm you in high levels.

### Driving Safety

Air bags do save lives, but you should always wear your seat belt when traveling regardless of how short your drive. When possible, purchase vehicles with air bags—they save lives. Be sure to know your road conditions and take caution when traveling in foul weather.

### Home Safety

Simple investments such as smoke detectors and fire extinguishers are a valuable asset to improving the safety of your home. Be sure you have a fire escape plan and that all family members know what to do in case of a house fire. To prevent falls, ensure that all stairways are clear of clutter and handrails are secure. The bathroom can be one of the most dangerous rooms in the house. Make sure that the bathtub has a slip free mat and be sure the temperature on the hot water thermostat is set so that the water is not too hot to reduce the risk of scalding.

### Sexual Health & Safety

A healthy sex life can contribute to overall good health and emotional well being. Regular sexual activity has been shown to decrease blood pressure and stress and reduce symptoms of depression.[23] It is important to incorporate sexual health into our lives as part of a healthy and happy personal relationship. Remember, that being sexually healthy also means that we avoid infections, illnesses and take personal responsibility to ensure that we protect ourselves and others, both emotionally and physically.

# Water Consumption

## Quench Your Thirst

In America, we take clean water for granted. So much so that we have begun drinking just about anything that is put into a plastic bottle and labeled "water". Poor water supplies and dirty water were the cause of the vast majority of illness and deaths before the turn of the century and in many parts of the world today, water borne disease is still the leading cause of death. In fact, the biggest public health action that accounted for raising the average age in America from 48 to 68, then from 68 to 70 was providing clean drinking water through chlorination and pasteurization of milk. Today, the number one health problem in Africa and many other countries is the inability to obtain clean drinking water. The bottom line, your body needs clean water and lots of it.

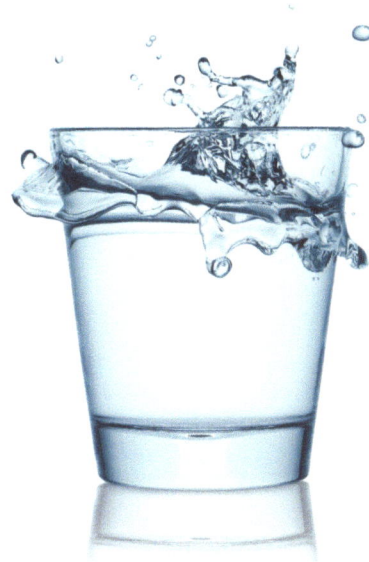

Mild to moderate dehydration plagues all of us. It is a busy world that we live in so we just do not take the time to drink enough clean water. Mild headaches, fatigue and muscle aches and back pain can all be caused by mild to moderate dehydration. The symptoms come on gradually and we live with them, until ultimately you go to your doctor to be fixed. The next thing you know you are taking a host of medications for something that could be fixed by just drinking water.

Yes! Water is a healthy part of your diet and should be consumed in recommended quantities daily. Increased water consumption is important when losing weight. But did you know that today some water can be dangerous to your health. Today many Americans drink bottled spring water. These spring waters contain additional minerals that sometimes in high quantities can actually make you sick. Clean water sources are simply H2O and not much else. Some bottled water contains minerals or mineral additives that can actually make you sick and cause an upset stomach. Your upset stomach may be caused from additional potassium and other added minerals in bottled spring waters. These added minerals and electrolytes can be very harmful for some individuals with certain medical problems.

So, clean water seems like a trivial matter, but as you can see it is not. Drink clean chlorinated drinking. If you choose to drink bottled water, then select water without minerals or electrolytes added and that comes from a reputable city water source. There are clean sources of bottled waters on the market-look for bottled water that is labeled purified (reverse osmosis) or from a public water source without added minerals and electrolytes like potassium. Some bottled water can have high levels of nitrites which can cause temporary sexual dysfunction.

# Mind Over Matter

## Your Brain Health - Keep It Healthy[24]

Your brain is the computer and the engine of your body. A well cared for brain slows the aging process! If your brain suffers then your body suffers in all respects, even down to your skin. Through the science of brain scanning techniques it is proven that you can actually improve your health through the health of your brain. To stay healthy and maintain optimal brain health here are some brain health tips to consider:

- Avoid toxins and substance abuse
- Avoid obesity – and large loads of carbohydrates
- Avoid brain trauma – head collisions (wear a safety helmet when appropriate)
- Avoid alcohol overuse and abuse – it's a toxin and doubles your chances of getting Alzheimer's
- Avoid things that decrease brain blood flow – like smoking and caffeine
- Avoid low levels of hormones – Estrogen/Testosterone – Thyroid and others
- Avoid prolonged stress and anxiety
- Recognize and treat depression – depression hurts your brain and overall health
- Chemotherapy kills brain cells so weigh the side effects depending on your cancer stage
- Avoid taking the flu vaccine from a multi-dose vial since these vials use thimerosal (thimerosal contains Mercury in very small amounts). If you take the flu vaccine then take it from single dose vials. The single-dose units are made without thimerosal as a preservative because they are intended to be opened and used only once. Additionally, the live-attenuated version of the vaccine (the nasal spray vaccine), is produced in single-dose units and does not contain thimerosal.

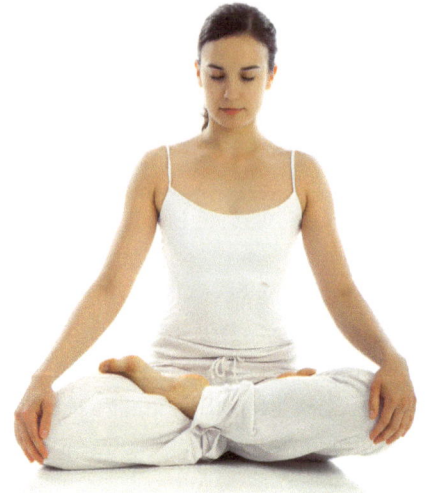

To ensure your brain is optimally performing and contributing to your good health engage and/or adopt the following health habits:

- Try to get a good night's rest - sleep at least 6 hours or more per day.
- Drastically decrease your alcohol intake.
- Loose excess weight – overweight and obesity leads to depression and dementia.
- Exercise to increase blood flow to your brain.
- Exercise your brain by reading, engaging in brain games like Sudoku, puzzles or other brain "teasers".
- Use food as medicine for your brain – eat right and decrease your carbohydrates
- Eat green leafy vegetables, nuts and berries, Omega 3 oils and drink green tea
- Take a good multivitamin that includes; Fish Oil, Vitamin D, Gingko, Vinpocetine, Huperzine, Acetyl L Carnitine.
- Meditate at least 15 minutes a day to relax your mind and restore your body.

# How To Interact With Your Doctor

## Helpful Tips You Should Know

**Doctors are people too.** They are busy, usually overworked and tired. Never hesitate to tell your doctor everything about what is bothering you including conditions with your in-laws, your marriage or whatever situations are stressing you. Why? Because stress causes many of the symptoms and conditions that you may be experiencing. Even the slightest "little thing" that you might forget to tell your doctor could be the one fact that can help with your diagnosis. Be honest and open with your doctor. Do not be embarrassed to talk about anything. In addition, tell your doctor if there are any barriers or problems that you may interfere with your care plan such as paying for medications or understanding his/her care directions.

**Don't ramble.** Make a list of the things you want to speak with your doctor about so that you can get to the point quickly. This really helps your doctor and maximizes the time you spend with him/her. It is difficult for some doctors to completely get all the information they need from you—so be prepared for your visit. Don't expect the doctor to read your mind or expect the doctor to come up with a diagnosis every time or even give you a prescription. In most instances your condition will not require a prescription. In fact, it is safer for you not to receive a prescription as most prescription medications have other side effects that can actually make you sicker. Drugs are not the solution to every health problem.

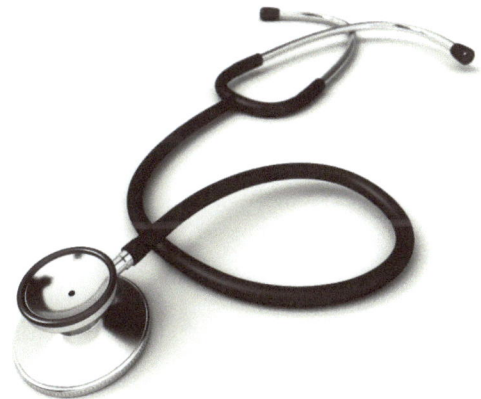

**Medicine is not a science.** Doctors do not have all the answers, so don't expect a precise answer all the time for what ails you. The vast majority of chronic disease is self induced. Think about your own behaviors and how they may be causing your problems; smoking, eating to many carbohydrates (over eating/over weight), the type of foods you eat and how you handle stress. Small, incremental lifestyle and behavior changes in any of these aspects of your life may resolve your problem without having to see a doctor.

**Never substitute a drug for a simple behavior change.** Unfortunately, many doctors in an attempt to satisfy their patients will tend to put you on a medication when a simple change in your health habits and behavior will make a difference. All drugs have side effects. Some side effects creep up on you and some are just outright deadly.

**Do not be afraid to ask why.** Always ask your doctor why he wants to do a certain test or prescribe a particular medication for you. If he doesn't take the time to explain, then find another doctor that will. Before you leave the doctor's office, make sure that you understand your condition, your instructions and how to take any prescribed medication. Use the internet to read about your condition. Don't depend solely on the doctor to get better. It's your body. Do what you need to get better, including changing your behaviors. If you're not sure about your diagnosis then seek another opinion. A second opinion is common and most doctors do not mind. It's your health-- make sure that you understand the risks associated with any recommended treatment and exactly why you have to have a procedure or surgery. Generally seek out the best doctor in your area. You may need to seek a specialist outside of your community. Get as much information on the doctor and hospital that you wish to use before you engage the system. Always ask questions and be sure to get answers.

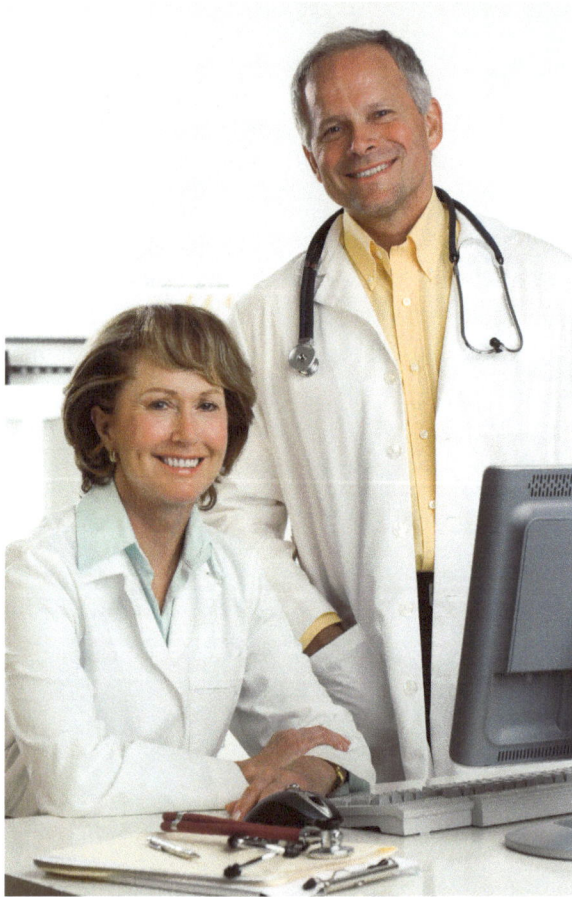

Don't be bashful about asking your doctor for a reduced fee for services. Since most doctors give big insurance companies a 30-50% discount it only makes sense that physicians offer similar discounts to conscientious healthcare consumers, especially if you have a high deductible health plan.

The Myth of Cholesterol and Heart Disease. There is no evidence that cholesterol or elevated cholesterol causes heart disease. The world population has been lead astray by physician and advertising opinions, that infer that controlling of your cholesterol will save you from heart disease. These opinions are simply NOT true. The US population spends over $10 billion dollars a year just on medications that "control" cholesterol. Many billions more are spent on testing and "fixing" the terrible side effects that these medications cause. There is a great body of evidence (known since the mid-seventies) that points to inflammation of the artery walls as the real cause of heart disease.[25]

Cholesterol is just an innocent bystander and this lipoprotein may actually be used by the body to repair damaged arterial walls. There can be several causes of inflammation in your body but the very diet that you have been told to eat, a diet low in fat and high in polyunsaturated fat combined with high sugar intake, is the biggest culprit of all. This diet can actually cause the inflammation in your arteries and then cholesterol begins to be deposited.

So, even if your cholesterol is low you can die of heart disease; something we have always known but simply discounted as unexplainable. You are encouraged to have this conversation with your doctor. Visit the following websites to download important industry information that speaks to the myth of cholesterol and heart disease.

http://www.simplicityhealthplan.com/files/downloads/articlesforthedownloadsite/what-really-causes-heart-disease.pdf

http://www.simplicityhealthplan.com/files/downloads/articlesforthedownloadsite/Cholesterol_Bloomberg_Article_2008.pdf

http://www.simplicityhealthplan.com/files/downloads/articlesforthedownloadsite/Cholesterol_HDL_NY_Times_5-2012.pdf

The widespread use of low dose aspirin, which works to decrease inflammation, actually does lower the rate of heart attacks. This simple relationship may indeed be a clue to solving the riddle of a diseased heart artery. Be sure to speak with your doctor on this important topic (people on blood thinners cannot use aspirin and should consult their doctor).

# Only You Can Improve Your Health

As a nurse of twenty years and a physician of thirty-four years and having spent the last 15 years of our careers focused on population health management, we can definitely say that we haven't been able to make anyone healthy except for those patients who are willing to be accountable and responsible for their own health. We both strongly believe in population health management and the power of prevention as one path that will lead the United States out of the current healthcare crisis. YOU must want to change your health and be empowered to do so through intrinsic motivation—meaning that your personal motivation to change comes from deep inside you. Good health will provide you the ultimate reward.

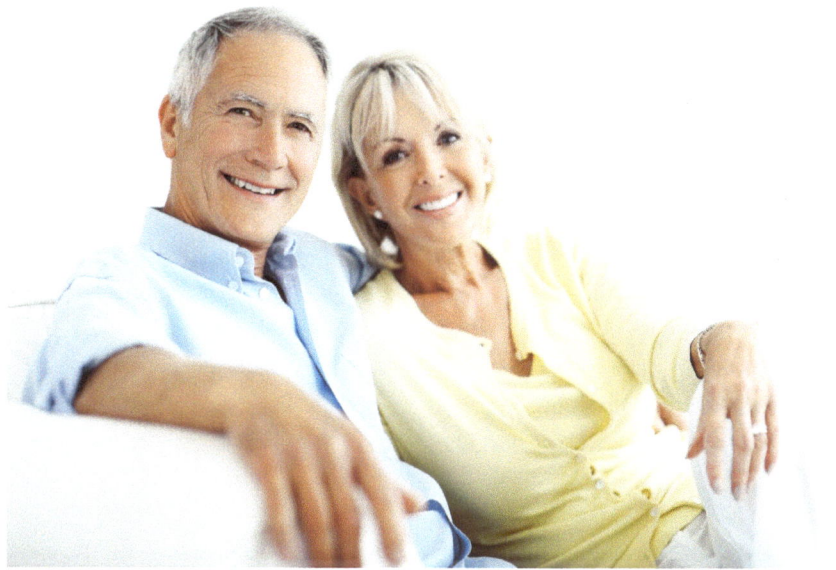

If you become accountable and responsible for your health, you will be able to achieve a sense of satisfaction in accomplishing your health goals. In addition, you will be saving a lot of money because you will not need to spend it on medications and other healthcare expenses.

Many employers are offing wellness programs to help keep their employees happy but these employers cannot fight this battle alone. They cannot make YOU healthy. YOU must want to change your health behaviors and lifestyles of your own accord, all of the wellness programs in the world will never reduce the expense associated with bad behavior. Adopting behaviors and lifestyles will truly lead to real risk reduction, overall good health and financial wellness.

Today, most individual's view their overall health as "good" regardless of the fact that their waist circumference is greater than forty inches and their blood pressure is 130/85mmHg. This is the group of people we like to call the healthy sick. The challenge is getting you to acknowledge that your health is not "so good" and to understand that YOU must become personally accountable and responsible for your health in order to achieve optimal well-being. This booklet provides you with the eight (8) essential steps to achieving a healthy and wealthy life. Read this booklet often and adopt the behavior change strategies we recommend to start yourself and your family on a road to wellness.

We understand that your life is busy; you're stressed with trying to balance a career and a family. This is EXACTLY the reason why you need to be as healthy as you can be. No one can make you healthy. YOU have what it takes, deep inside, to make a change. Don't delay another day. Be accountable, be responsible, take care of yourself and make yourself healthy, happy and wealthy!

# Financial Wellness

## Your Health Choices Can Help You Save for Your Future (Health2Cash™ App)

Today, individuals do not have significant disposable income to set aside for retirement. The general level of confidence among individuals regarding their ability to afford retirement is at an all-time low.[26] In most cases, individuals simply do not know where to find the additional income to set aside for retirement.

Americans spend $2.5 trillion dollars on healthcare, twice what the rest of the world does and yet we rank 17th in overall health. We estimate that Americans are wasting about $200 billion a year in unwarranted healthcare and another $600 billion in healthcare that would otherwise be unnecessary if they simply changed their lifestyles and health behaviors.

This booklet has provided you the eight fundamental health elements to healthier living. It is imperative that you bridge the gap between physical health and financial wellness to achieve financial security for your future.

It has been reported that healthcare related expenses will increase throughout your retirement. It is estimated that a relatively healthy couple will need to have saved over $250,000.00 just to address unreimbursed healthcare expenses throughout their retired lives.[27]

By making an effort to improve your lifestyles and health behaviors today, you will not only be working toward a better quality of life but you will be establishing the ability to increase your personal wealth and look forward to a wealthy retirement.

Let's face it, without good health your ability to accumulate sufficient wealth for retirement becomes very unlikely. How can you predict what your health is costing you in real dollars? Use the Health Index Calculator, it is that simple! The Health Index Calculator will help you forecast and visualize your savings potential. The Health Index Calculator is only a best estimate of potential savings and is meant to be used as a guideline to help you save.

The Health Index Calculator is an innovative, easy-to-use web-based application available to you on the StayFit Plan platform (ask your employer) that allows you to gauge **real** dollar savings that can be achieved through simple health behavior change. Ultimately, these savings can be used to fund you retirement by investing those savings into your Health Savings Account (HSA) or 401K in order to achieve financial security.
The Health Index Calculator calculates and estimates the everyday economic impact of eight distinct health behaviors that impact the majority of your income and then forecasts significant economic savings based on the health improvement goals you determine.

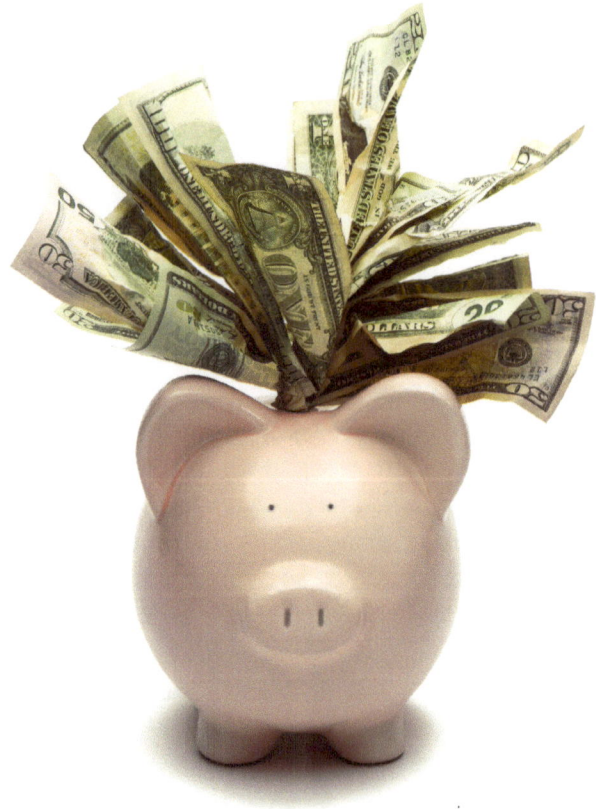

# Financial Wellness (continued)

You simply adjust the calculator "sliders" to your desired future health (goal) to visualize your estimated cash savings. Embedded health resources help you learn how to change the desired behavior to get you on a path to health and wealth quickly. The calculator will automatically send you Alerts that serve as a reminder to help you keep the new goals that you set within the calculator. Remember that saving your payroll dollars before tax into your retirement accounts saves you a considerable amount of cash (not paid as taxes) and can be looked at as an immediate 30-50% return.

Be on the lookout for the Health Index Calculator™ App, Health2Cash™ through the Apple® I-Tunes site or as an Android App. The App offers a fun and interactive approach to realizing the economic impact of your health behavior changes.

# Stay Fit For Life

## Diet and Exercise Plans

The benefits of physical activity are tremendous to mind, body and spirit. Today, most Americans do not get enough physical activity. The inclusion of physical activity in your daily life is essential to overall good physical and mental health. Individuals who include at least 30 minutes of moderate physical activity have been shown to decrease or eliminate many symptoms associated with certain chronic disease. Stress, depression and digestive problems are minimized as exercise reduces daily tension and promotes a better digestive process. Your skin, the largest organ of your body, becomes healthier and muscle tone is revitalized improving endurance and core strength with sustainable exercise. Physical activity promotes improved cardiovascular function and better blood circulation. Physical fitness has a positive impact on your mental health and generally results in improved self-esteem as you can visualize a healthier and leaner you. You may find that you sleep better adding to your vitality. Finally, and what most people already know is that engaging in physical activity increases the number of calories your body burns for energy. If your body burns more calories than you are ingesting you will maintain or lose weight. Thirty minutes a day is such a small commitment for something that will bring you better health and well-being. The four most common physical activity programs that are easy to do and don't require any extra money for equipment or memberships are; walking, jogging, swimming and bicycling.

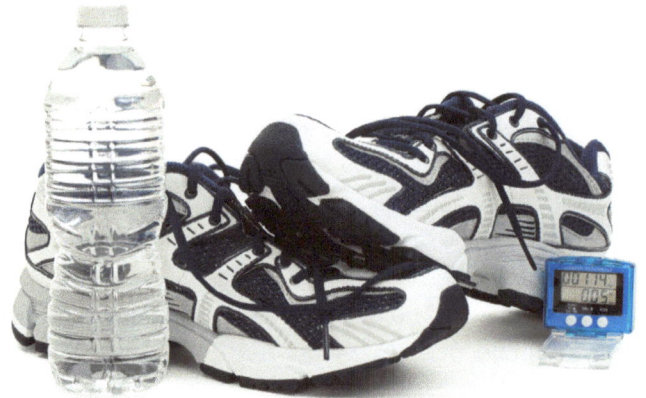

Weight loss and weight management is not easy. After all, the average portion size of foods in restaurants has more that doubled over the past 10 years and the "more is better" mentality has created a society of Americans with growing waistlines. The following behavior modifications are meant to be guidelines that you can adopt and may help you change the way you interact with food to achieve your weight loss goals.

- Eat slowly. Put your fork down between each bite and sip some water this will allow your brain time to recognize that it has been fed.
- When you are hungry ask yourself if you're truly hungry or are you craving food because you are bored? Drink a full glass of water and engage in an activity to distract your hunger. If you're still hungry then have a small healthy snack such as celery sticks or carrot sticks.
- If you choose to eat out look for low calorie, low fat entrees. Since portion sizes are so large you may want to order just one entrée and share it or if you're alone just order an appetizer. Avoid "all you can eat" restaurants and fast food chains.

The StayFit™ Plan has included a sample diet and exercise planner that you can print and customize to meet your specific needs. In addition you have access to a wide range of diet and exercise tools, resources and programs as part of the StayFit™ Plan. You can access these programs by clicking on the MyHealthCenter on the StayFit™ Plan website www.simplicityhealthplans.com. You can chat with a trainer, start an exercise blog, track your diet or get general exercise tips to help keep you motivated. Use your StayFit™ Plan Discount Program package for a variety of health and wellness discounts including diet and fitness discounts. So be sure to log on today!

*Note: Always consult with your healthcare provider before you begin a diet and exercise program.*

# Sample Workout and Exercise Plan

**Date:**    /    /      **Start Time:**    :    am/pm    **End Time:**    :    am/pm

| | |
|---|---|
| Scale Weight: | |
| Body Mass Index: | |
| Fitness Goal: | |
| Sleep (HRS/night) | |

BMI = (Weight in Pounds / Height in Inches x Height in Inches)) x 703

## Exercise Focus (Circle all that applies):

Whole body  I  Legs  I  Chest  I Back  I Shoulders I Arms I Abdominal I Other (specify): _____

## Cardiovascular Training:

| Exercise Type: | Calories Burned or Distance: | Time: |
|---|---|---|
| | | |
| | | |
| | | |

## Strength Training (All exercises should be done bilaterally):

| Exercise: | Sets: | Reps: | Rest Period: | Notes: |
|---|---|---|---|---|
| **Upper Body:** | | | | |
| Bent over row | 3 - 4 | 12 | 10 - 15 sec | |
| Back extensions | 3 - 4 | 12 | 10 - 15 sec | |
| Chest press | 3 - 4 | 12 | 10 - 15 sec | |
| Push ups | 3 - 4 | 12 | 10 - 15 sec | |
| Standing bicep curls | 3 - 4 | 12 | 10 - 15 sec | |
| Overhead tricep extension | 3 - 4 | 12 | 10 - 15 sec | |
| Side raises | 3 - 4 | 12 | 10 - 15 sec | |
| **Abdominal:** | | | | |
| Torso twist with bar | 2 - 3 | 30 | Hold 20 sec each side | |
| Sit ups | 3 - 4 | 15 | 10 - 15 sec | |
| Leg raises | 2 - 3 | 12 | 10 - 15 sec | |
| Bicycle/leg scissors | 2 - 3 | 12 | 10 - 15 sec | |

- Select the entire circuit plan or choose a section of the plan or select four (4) exercises for each training session; rotating exercises until you have performed all.
- Be sure to use the StayFit™ Plan exercise tools, resources and programs located on the MyHealthCenter on the StayFit™ Plan website at www.simplicityhealthplans.com.
- This training plan is a recommendation only and is not meant to be all inclusive or prescriptive. Always check with your personal healthcare provider before beginning an exercise program.

# Sample Meal Progress Plan

**Date:** / /     **Start BMI:**     **End**ing BMI:

*Always check with your personal health care provider before beginning any weight management program.*

| Plan | Actual |
|---|---|
| Total portions of protein: **6** | Total portions of protein: |
| Total portions of carbohydrates: **6** | Total portions of carbohydrates: |
| Total glasses (8 oz) of water: **10** | Total glasses (8 oz) of water: |
| Exercise: **30 - 45 minutes moderate intensity** | Exercise: |

| Plan: | Actual: |
|---|---|
| Meal 1 | Meal 1 |
| ☐ am ☐ pm | ☐ am ☐ pm |
| Meal 2 | Meal 2 |
| ☐ am ☐ pm | ☐ am ☐ pm |
| Meal 3 | Meal 3 |
| ☐ am ☐ pm | ☐ am ☐ pm |
| Meal 4 | Meal 4 |
| ☐ am ☐ pm | ☐ am ☐ pm |
| Meal 5 | Meal 5 |
| ☐ am ☐ pm | ☐ am ☐ pm |
| Meal 6 | Meal 6 |
| ☐ am ☐ pm | ☐ am ☐ pm |

Notes: _____

_____

_____

# References
## Health and Wellness Guide

1. Centers for Disease Control and Prevention. http://www.cdc.gov/chronicdisease/resources/publications/AAG/chronic.htm

2. The Council of State Governments. (2006) Costs of Chronic Disease. What are States Facing?

3. United States Preventive Service Task Force. Adult Preventive Screening Guidelines.

4. Ogden, C. et al. (2012) The Prevalence of Obesity in the United States, 2009-2010. NCHS Data Brief, No.83, January 2012.

5. Centers for Disease Control and Prevention. Overweight and Obesity, the Health Consequences. http://www.cdc.gov/obesity/causes/health.html

6. American College of Sports Medicine.

7. The American Cancer Society. Stay Away from Tobacco. http://www.cancer.org/Healthy/StayAwayfromTobacco/index?ssSourceSiteId=null

8. United States Preventive Service Task Force. Adult Preventive Screening Guidelines. http://www.uspreventiveservicestaskforce.org/adultrec.htm

9. United States Department of Agriculture. www.myplate.gov

10. American Diabetic Association.

11. The Portion Plate. http://www.theportionplate.com/loss.html

12. The American Heart Association. Managing Your Blood Pressure with a Heart-Healthy Diet. http://www.heart.org/HEARTORG/Conditions/HighBloodPressure/PreventionTreatmentofHighBloodPressure/ManagingBlood-Pressure-with-a-Heart-Healthy-Diet_UCM_301879_Article.jsp

13. United States Department of Agriculture. Food and Nutrition Information Center. http://iom.edu/Activities/Nutrition/SummaryDRIs/~/media/Files/Activity%20Files/Nutrition/DRIs/RDA%20and%20AIs_Vitamin%20and%20Elements.pdf

14. Centers for Disease Control and Prevention. Overweight and Obesity.

15. The Obesity Society. What is Obesity? http://www.obesity.org/resources-for/what-is-obesity.htm?qh=YToyOntpOjA7czozOiJibWkiO2k6MTtzOjQ6ImJtaXMiO30%3D

16. Tuah. N. et (2011)Transtheoretical model for dietary and physical exercise modification in weight loss management for overweight and obese adults. http://www.ncbi.nlm.nih.gov/pubmed/21975777

17. Wikipedia. Yo-yo effect. http://en.wikipedia.org/wiki/Yo-yo_effect

18. John Hopkins Medical Center. The Risks of Physical Inactivity. http://www.hopkinsmedicine.org/healthlibrary/conditions/adult/cardiovascular_diseases/risks_of_physical_inactivity_85,P00218/

19. Donnelly, J. et al. (2009) Medicine & Science in Sports & Exercise: Appropriate Physical Activity Intervention Strategies for Weight Loss and Prevention of Weight Regain for Adults. Volume 41, Issue 2, pp 459-471.

20. American College of Sports Medicine.

21. The Health Status of the United States Workforce. (2007) Findings from the National Health and Nutrition Examination Survey (NHANES) 1999-2002 and the National Health Interview Survey (NHS) 2005.

22. The American Cancer Society. Stay Away from Tobacco. http://www.cancer.org/Healthy/StayAwayfromTobacco/index?ssSourceSiteId=null

23. WebMD. The 10 Surprising Benefits of Sex. http://www.webmd.com/sex-relationships/features/10-surprising-health-benefits-of-sex

24. Amen. Daniel G., M.D. Change Your Brain Change Your Body.

25. myscienceacademy.org (August, 2012) http://myscienceacademy.org/2012/08/19/world-renown-heart-surgeon-speaks-out-on-what-really-causes-heart-disease/

26. 2012 Retirement Confidence Survey conducted by the Employees Benefit Research Institute (EBRI) and Matthew Greenwald & Associates, Inc.

27. Funding Savings needed for Health Expenses for Persons Eligible for Medicare. EBRI Issue Brief, December 2010.

*Disclaimer:* Simplicity Health Plans was interested in learning if the information in this booklet was a helpful and educational resource and if prospective readers would find this guide valuable. To aid in this effort, Simplicity Health Plans conducted a focus group with healthcare consumer's 27-61 years of age to solicit qualitative feedback and recommendations based on the information provided to them in the guide. Overall feedback was overwhelmingly positive and focus group recommendations were considered and appropriately incorporated into the final version of the guide.

Notes: _____

**Notes:** _____

_____

_____

_____

_____

_____

_____

_____

_____

_____

_____

_____

_____

_____

_____

_____

_____

_____

_____

_____

_____

_____

_____

_____

_____

_____

_____

_____

_____

# About the Authors

## Gregory J. Hummer, M.D.

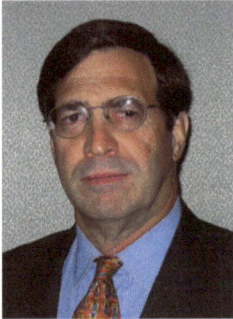

Dr. Hummer is Chairman and CEO of Simplicity Health Plans, founder of a national group of emergency centers called MED Center and most recently, the founder of Fortune Health, Ltd. and Health2Cash.Net. His career includes 30 years as a Cleveland trauma surgeon after training at the Cleveland Clinic Hospital as well as 3 years at the NASA Lewis Research Center where he served as the Director of Medical Screening. He has spent the last 32 years taking care of patients, developing successful healthcare companies and creating innovative healthcare software platforms to solve the vexing complexities, out-of-control costs, burdens and inefficiencies that are associated with today's American healthcare system.

Dr. Hummer is committed to helping individuals become healthy and wealthy by changing their health behaviors through consumerism solutions. He coauthored this informational guide to help our readers navigate through all of the nonsense that has been published about how to achieve good health. Most Americans do not realize that there are simple, easy solutions to staying healthy. The bottom line is that nobody is going to change your health except YOU! Read this guide today to learn how easy it is to get started on your way to achieving good health.

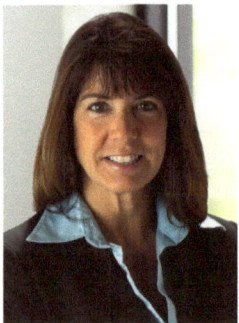

## Lisa M. Holland, RN, MBA

Lisa Holland has been in the healthcare industry for over 18 years and has held senior level positions for some of the largest healthcare organizations in the United States.

Lisa is an accomplished nurse and business development professional with a superior healthcare skill set that includes benefit plan design, population health management, clinical data analysis, marketing and clinical product development.

Lisa's passion, strength and knowledge are in primary prevention and wellness. Her professional objective is to use her knowledge and expertise to empower individuals to become responsible healthcare consumers and to achieve optimal health and well-being.

As coauthor, it was Lisa's objective to create a common sense health and wellness guide that offers simple strategies and solutions to help individuals achieve good health. This guide helps individuals understand that small incremental changes and appropriate choices can have a huge impact on personal health.

www.ingramcontent.com/pod-product-compliance
Lightning Source LLC
Chambersburg PA
CBHW060842270326
41933CB00002B/177